The Booger that Escaped

Written and Illustrated By:
Moment Johnson

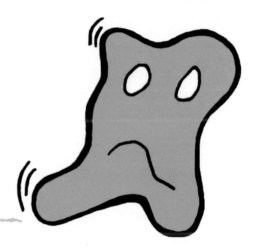

Lost Truth Press

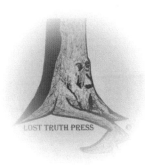

Lost Truth Press

ISBN - 13: 978-0-9882021-6-0
ISBN - 10: 0988202166

Other Books by Moment Johnson

The lost Piece

Little Caterpillar's Dilemma

I'm a Platypus

Ancient Giants of the Black Hills

Spike Becomes a Daddy

The Earth Keeps Spinning, but Never Gets Dizzy

Please Visit

www.losttruthpress.com

To all the curious kids who ask why?
about anything and everything.
"Why are you getting a tissue?"
"Because a booger is trying to escape from my nose."
And so this book was formed.

Somewhere deep inside a little girl's nostril ...

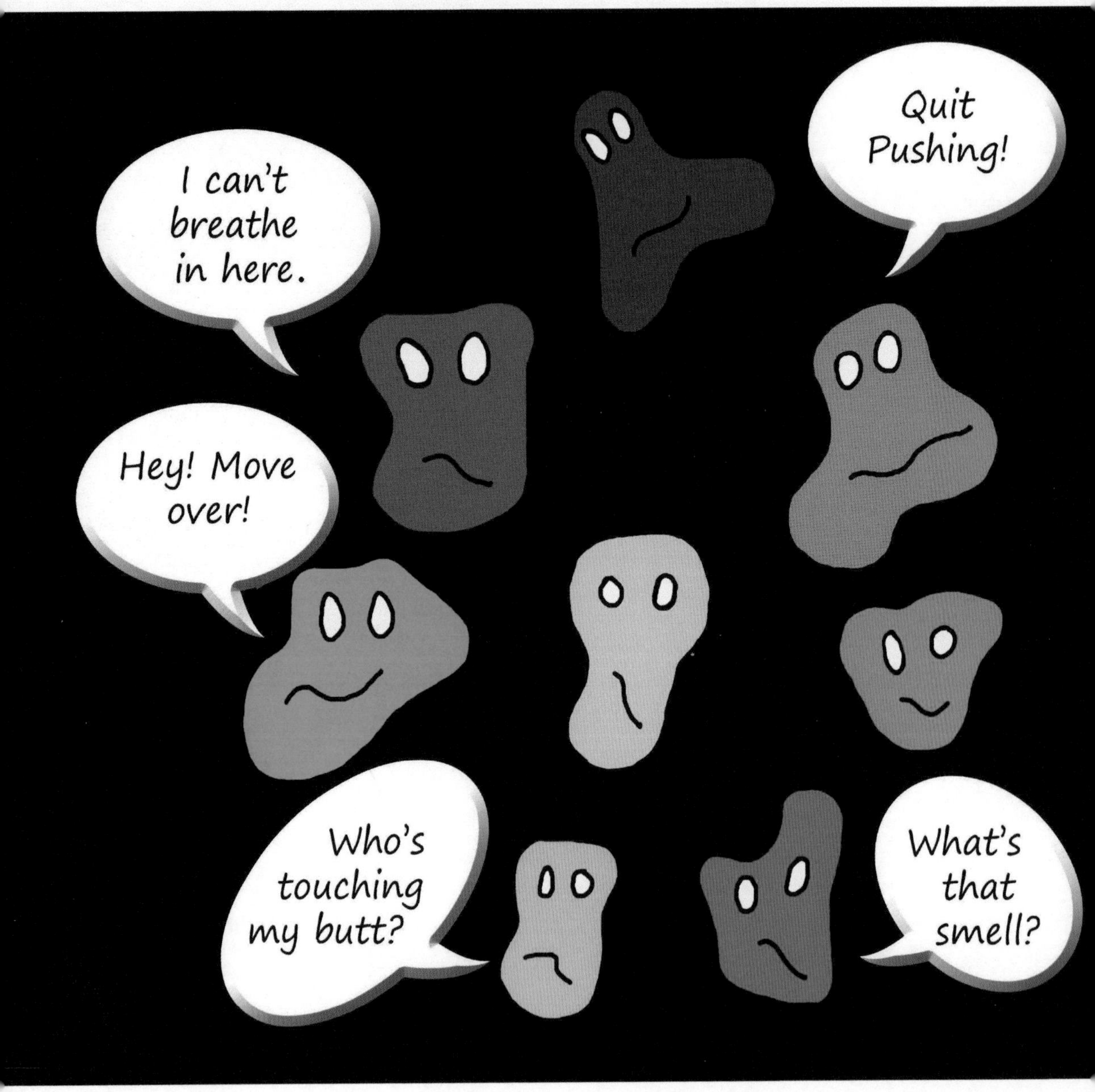
I can't breathe in here.
Quit Pushing!
Hey! Move over!
Who's touching my butt?
What's that smell?

... a colony of boogers began to gather.

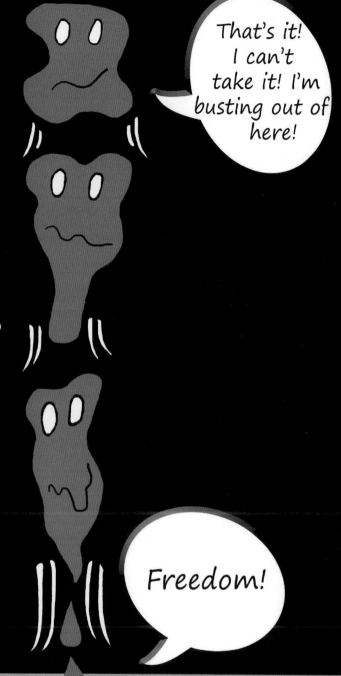

Then one of the
oogey, googey,
boogeys
began to melt.
Transforming into
snot, it dripped
out of the girl's
nose and down
her lip.

That's it! I can't take it! I'm busting out of here!
Freedom!

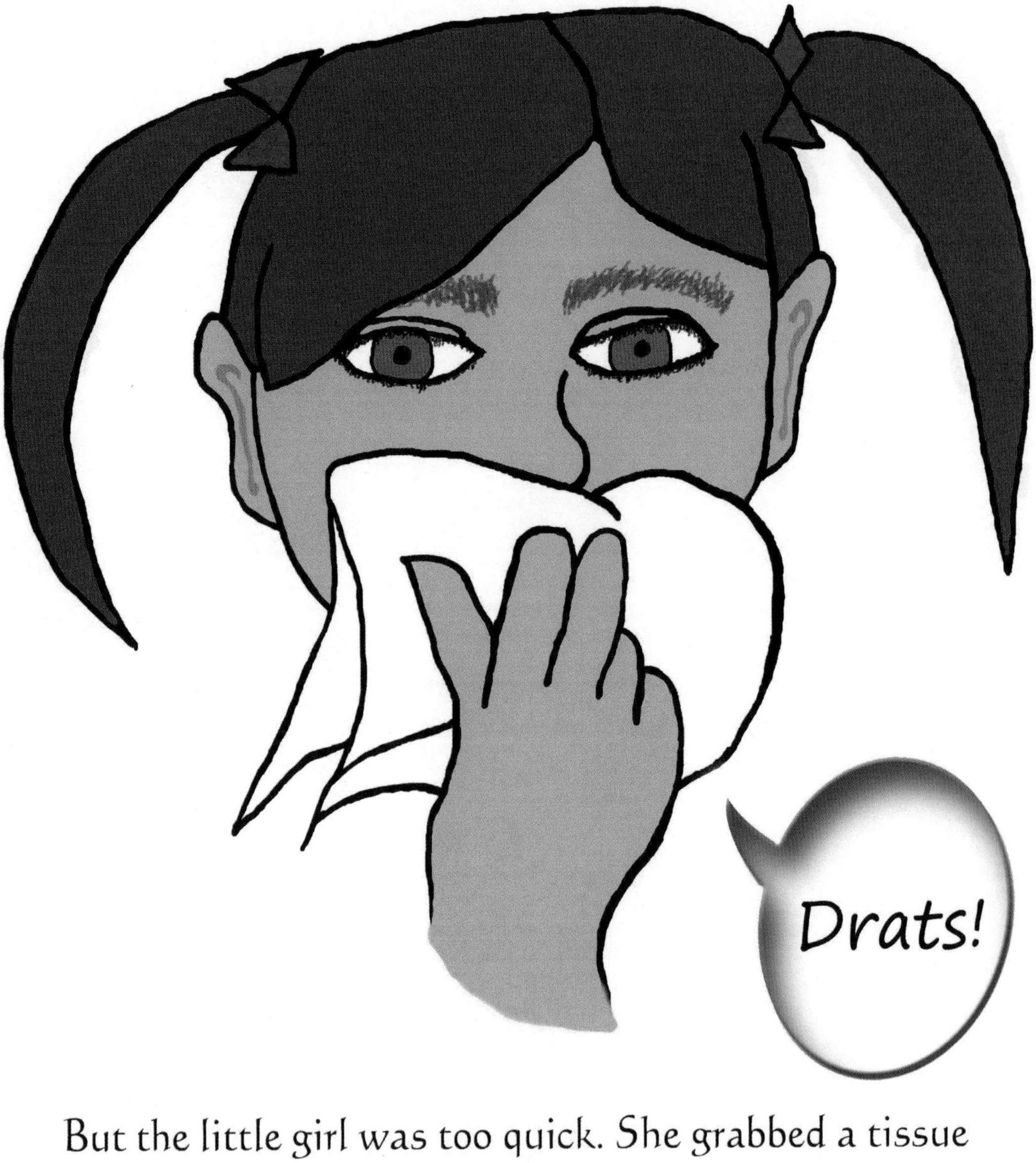
Drats!

But the little girl was too quick. She grabbed a tissue and wiped the ookey, yookey mucus away.

Back inside the nasal cavity...

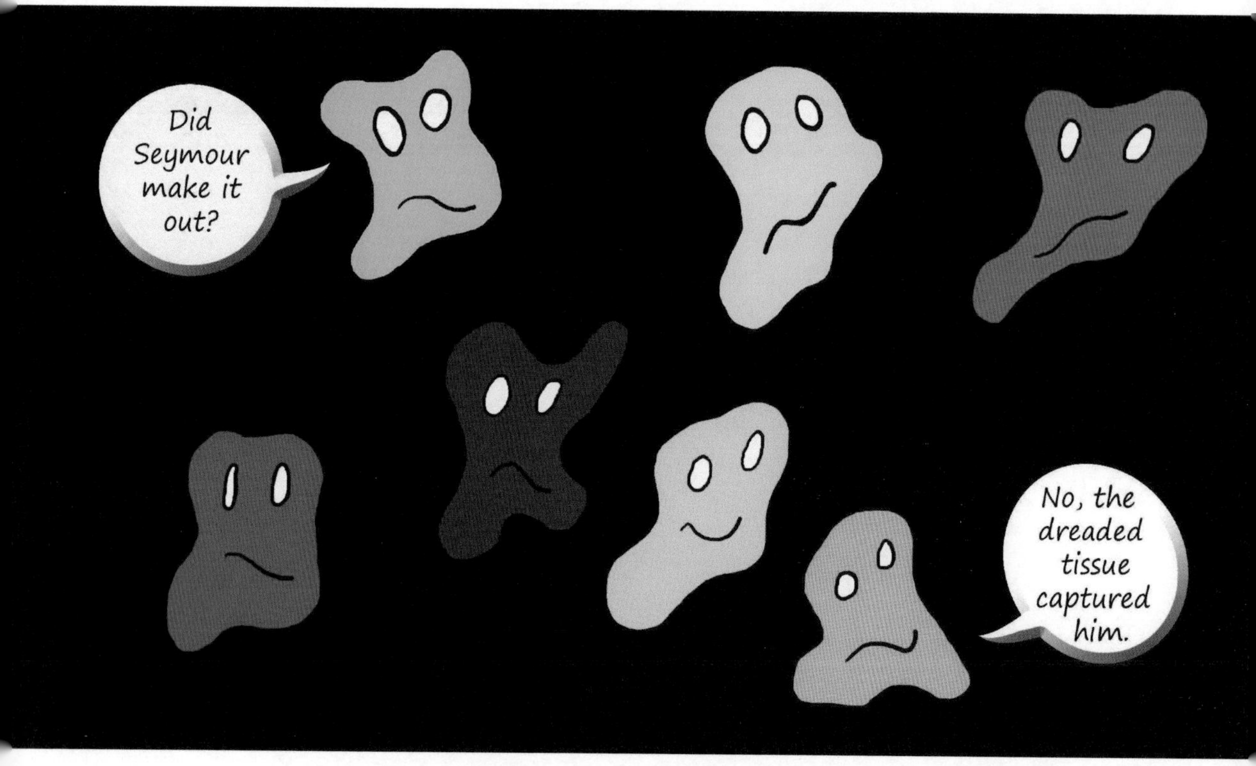
Did Seymour make it out?
No, the dreaded tissue captured him.

...over population was becoming a problem.

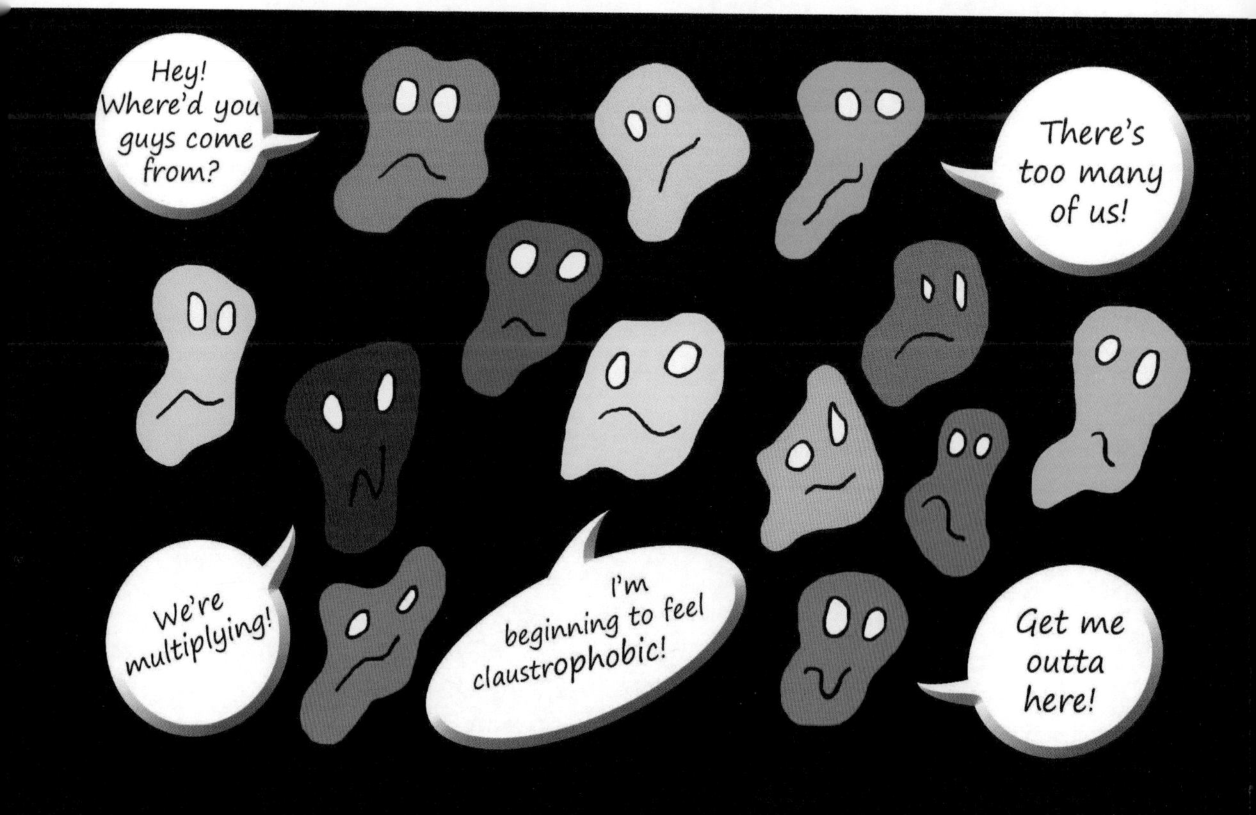
Hey! Where'd you guys come from?
There's too many of us!
We're multiplying!
I'm beginning to feel claustrophobic!
Get me outta here!

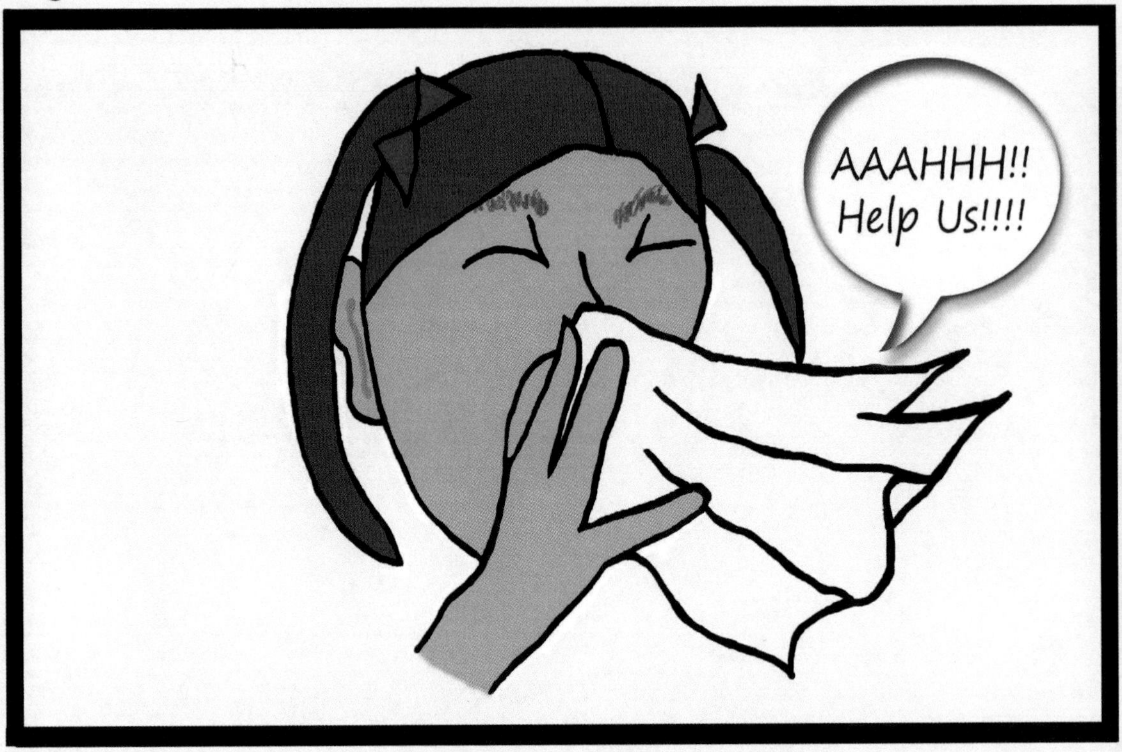
AAAHHH!!
Help Us!!!!

The little girl knew just what to do. She blasted those mutating nose goblins into a kleenex. Then tossed them into the garbage - gone forever.

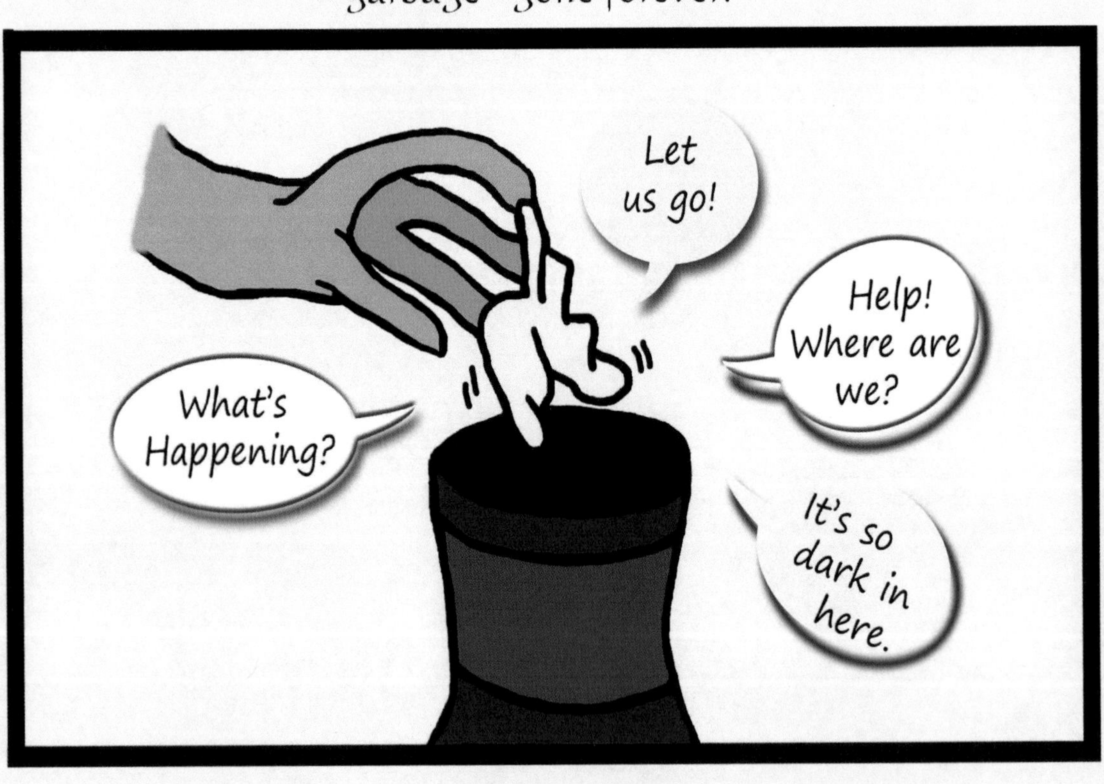
Let us go!
Help! Where are we?
What's Happening?
It's so dark in here.

Back at Booger Headquarters...

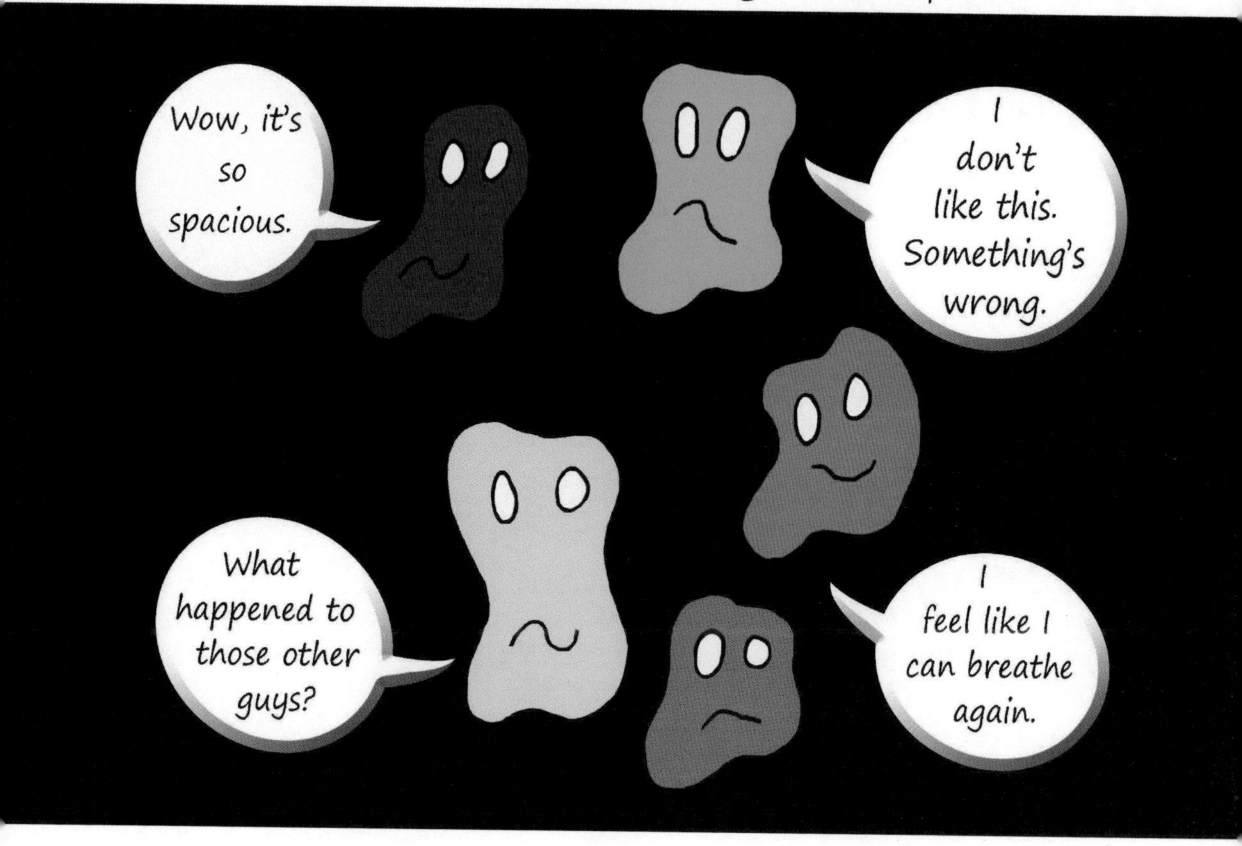
Wow, it's so spacious.
I don't like this. Something's wrong.
What happened to those other guys?
I feel like I can breathe again.

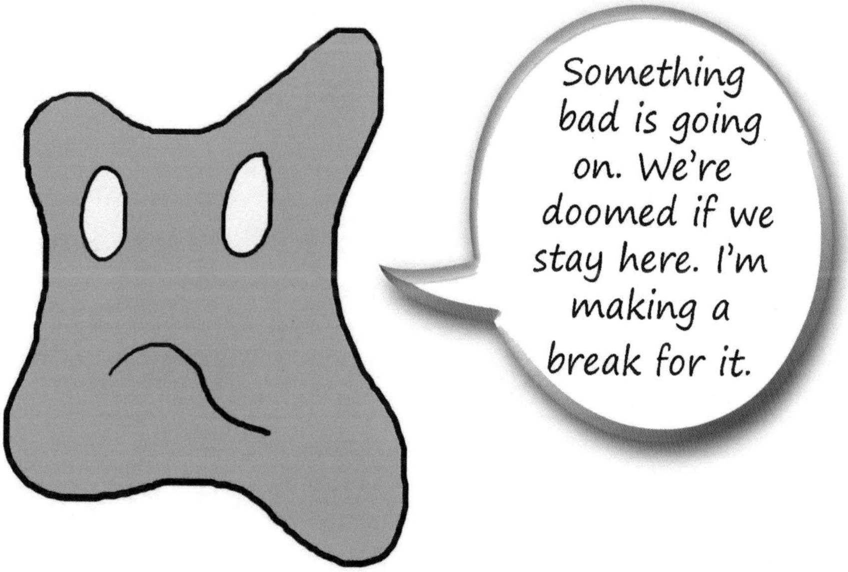
Something bad is going on. We're doomed if we stay here. I'm making a break for it.

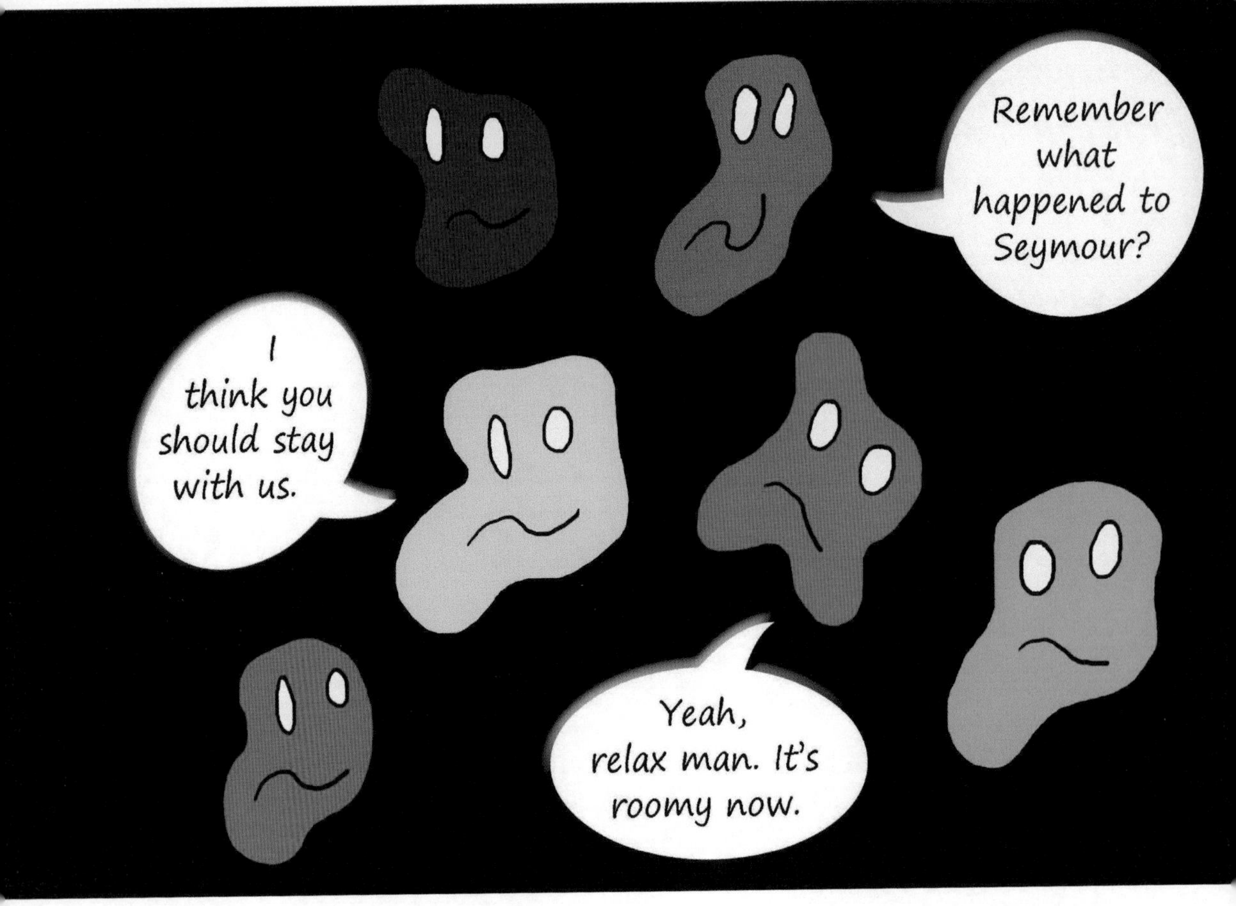
Remember what happened to Seymour?
I think you should stay with us.
Yeah, relax man. It's roomy now.

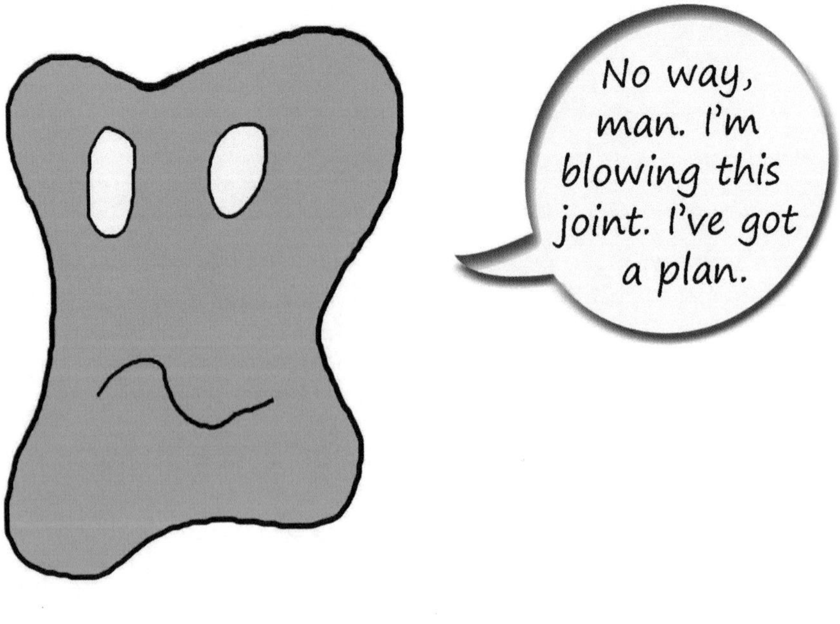
No way, man. I'm blowing this joint. I've got a plan.

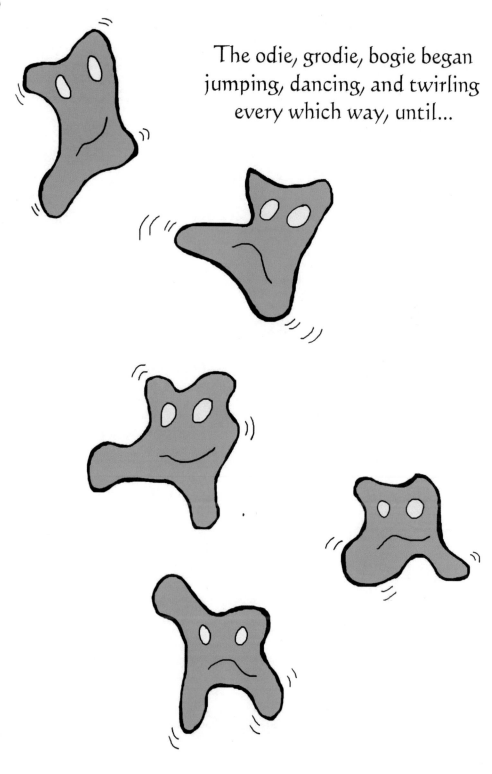

The odie, grodie, bogie began jumping, dancing, and twirling every which way, until...

AH

AH

AH

CHOO!!!

Whoopee!!
I'm Free!!

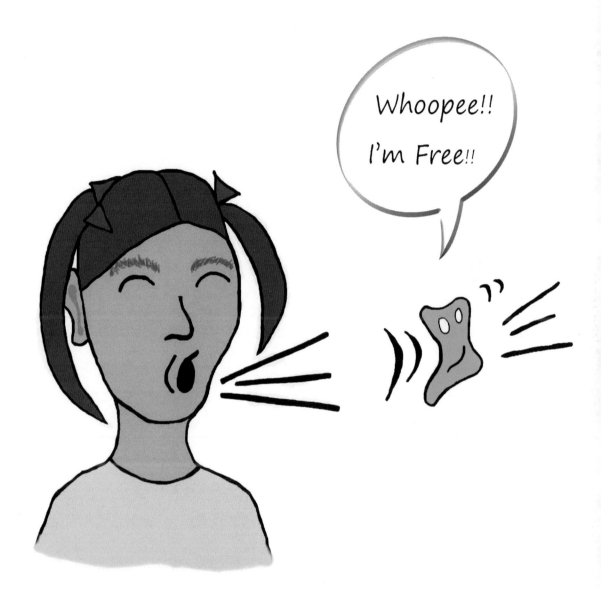

The grimey, blimey, slime ball shot straight out of the little girl's nose and landed on the unsuspecting hand of an innocent bystander.

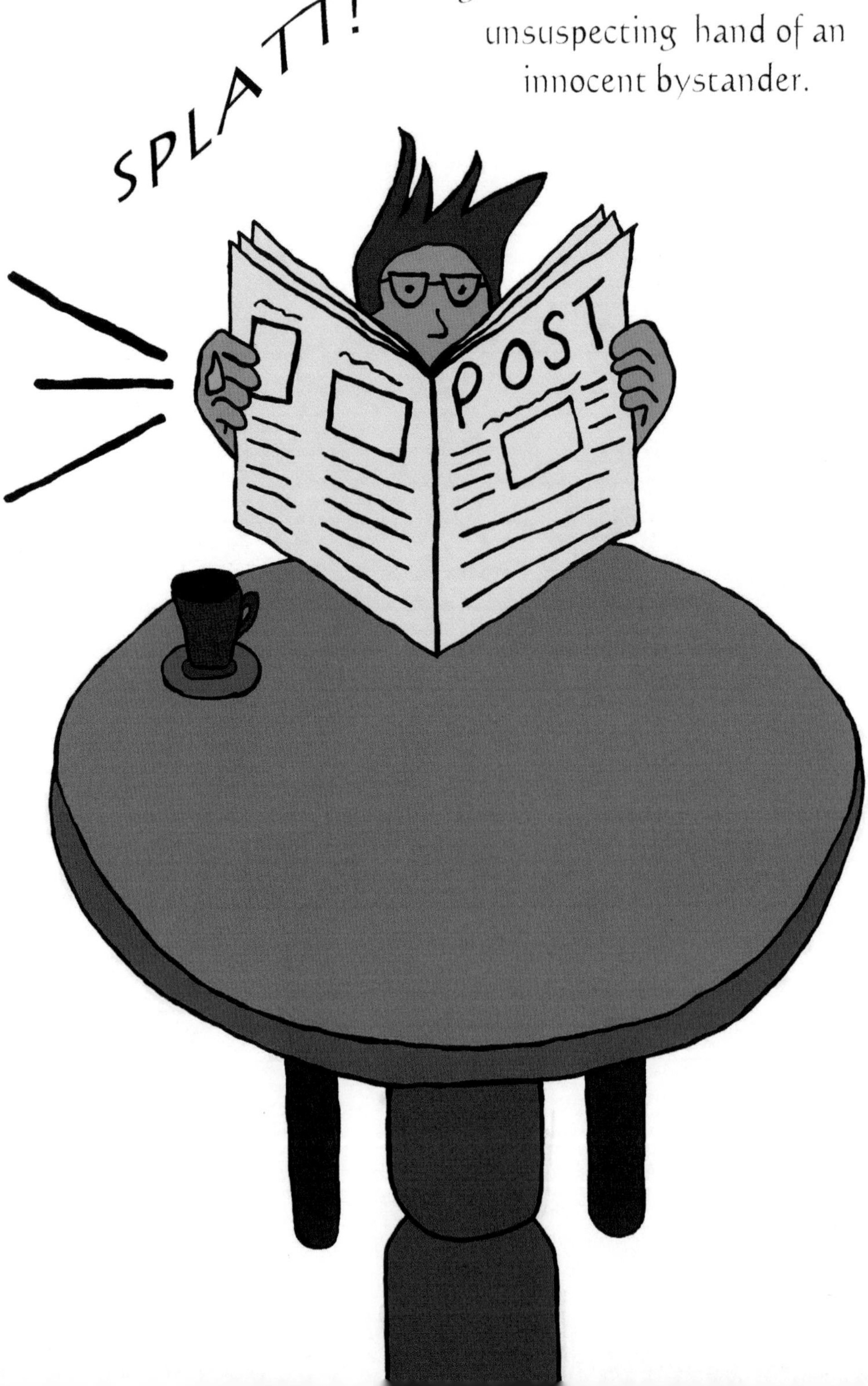
SPLATT!
POST

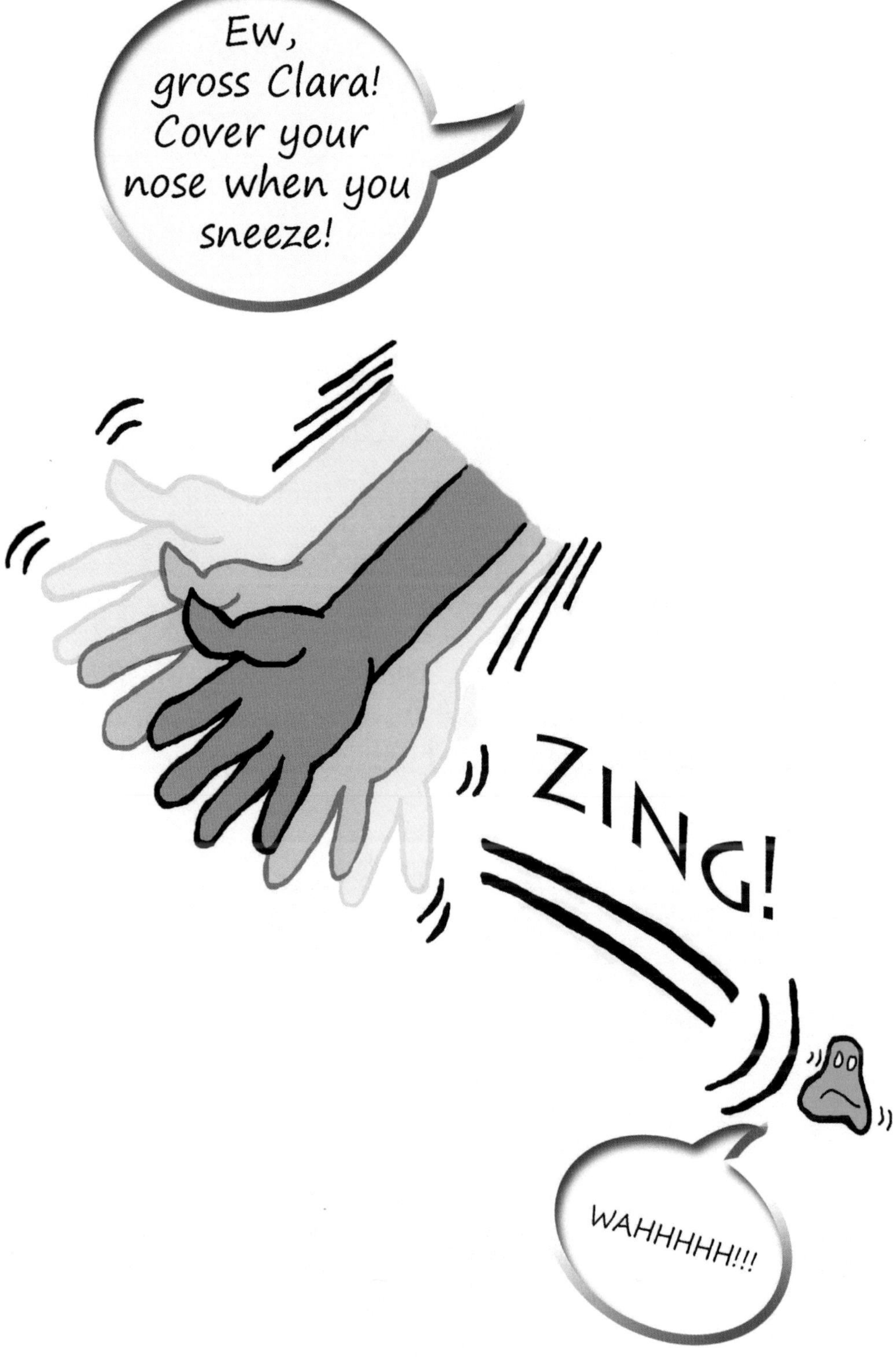
Ew,
gross Clara!
Cover your
nose when you
sneeze!
ZING!
WAHHHHH!!!

Fearing for his life, the snotball took off running across the table, leaving a trail of slick, slobbery slime behind him.

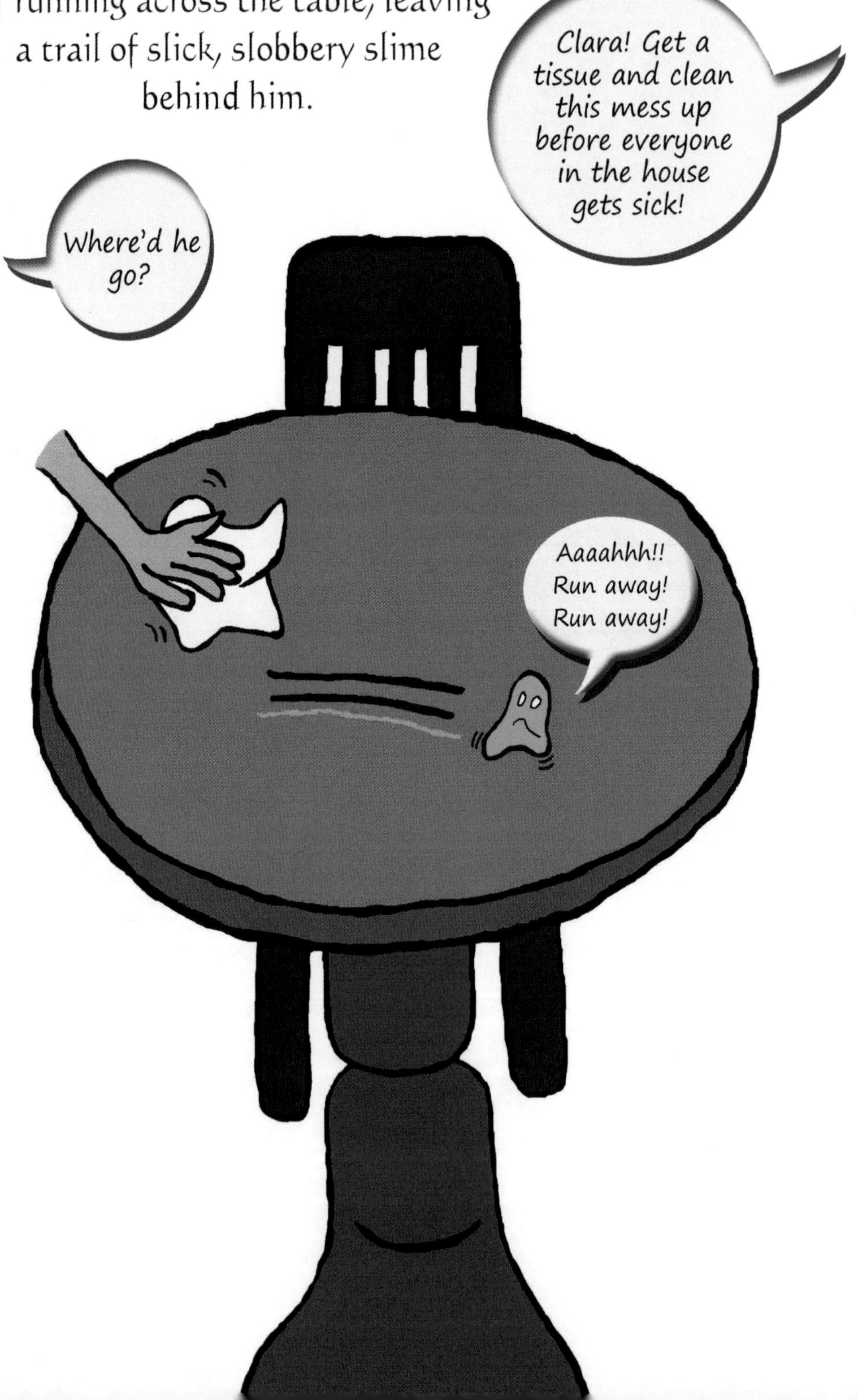
Clara! Get a tissue and clean this mess up before everyone in the house gets sick!
Where'd he go?
Aaaahhh!! Run away! Run away!

The sicky-icky, green and drippy, boogey leapt from the table, raced across the kitchen floor, over the carpet, and ducked behind the couch.

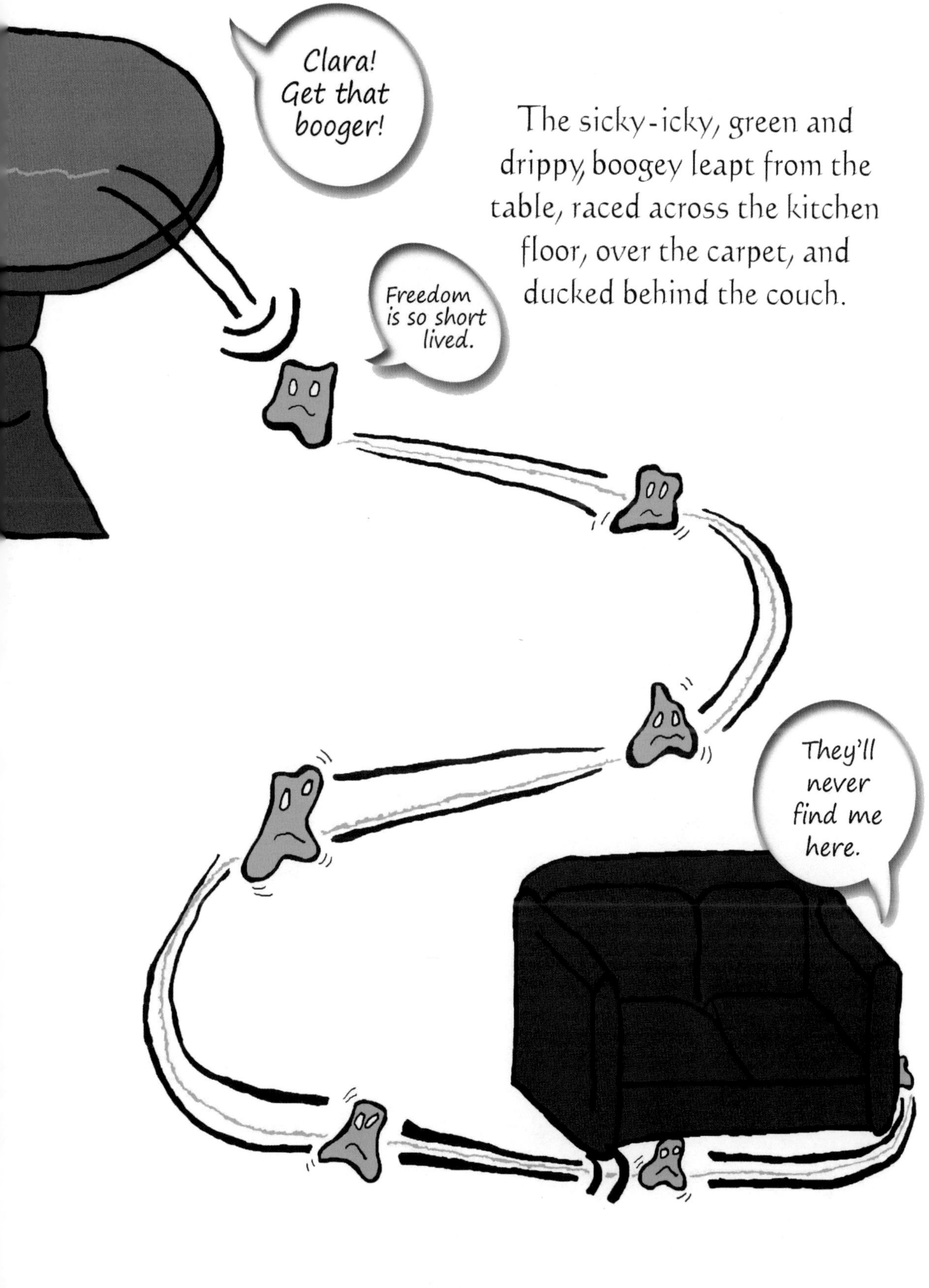
Clara! Get that booger!
Freedom is so short lived.
They'll never find me here.

Clara followed the trail of glistening, sickening, yellow and greening, ooey, gooey, mess.

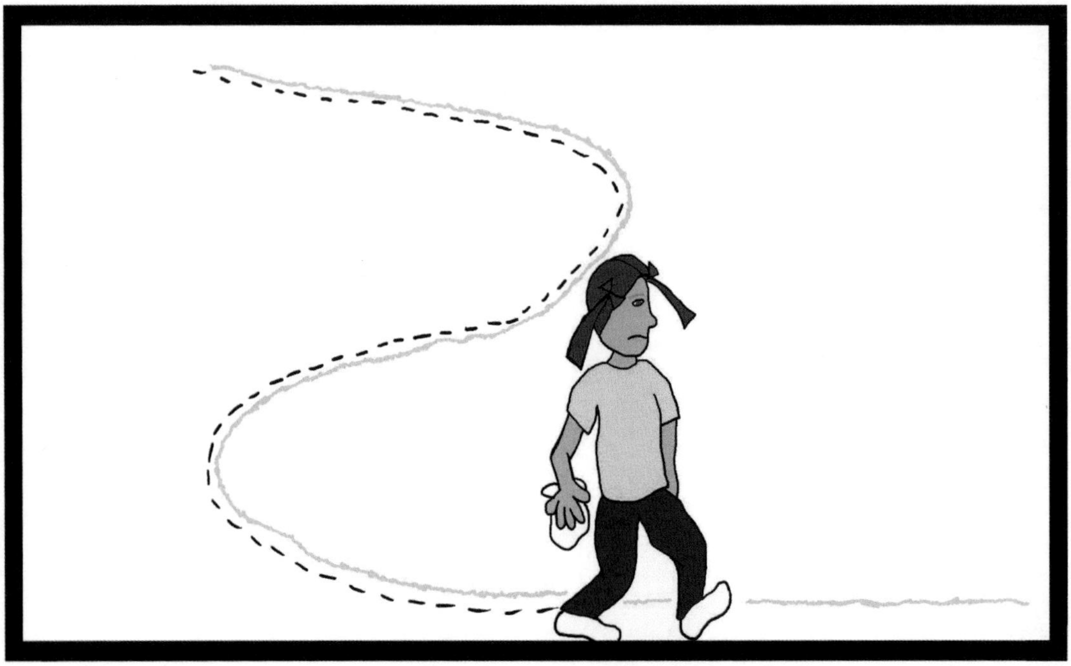

Zig-zagging across the house, she found that sneaky little booger hiding behind the couch.

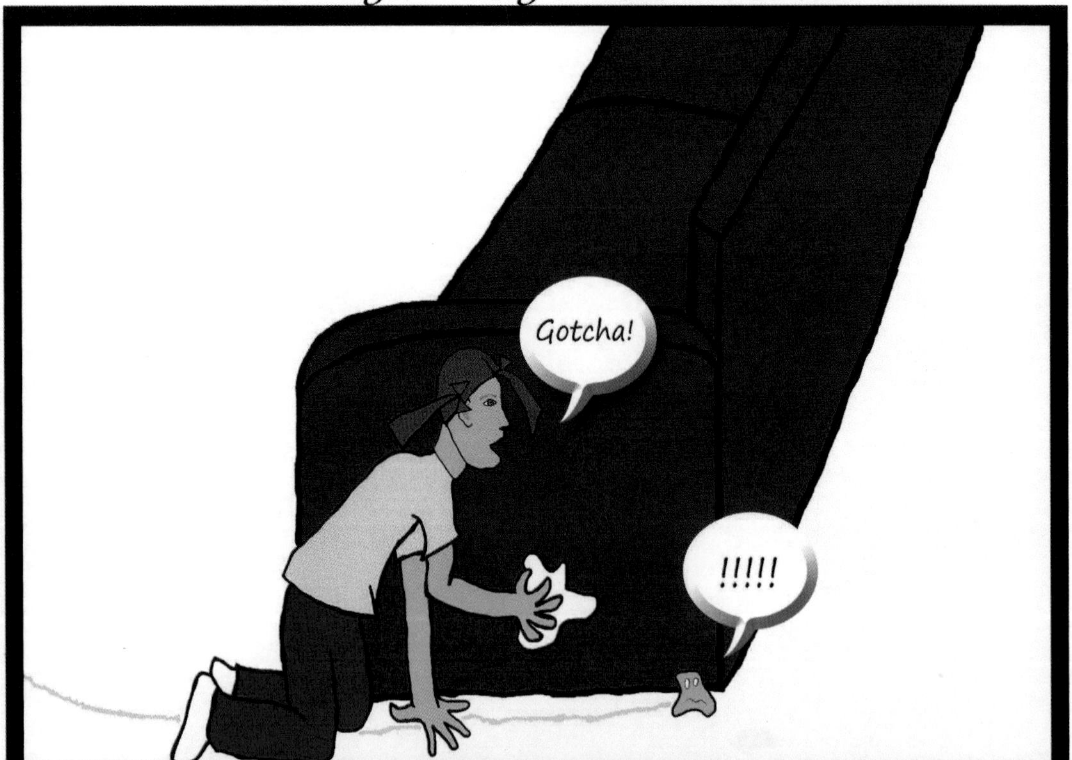
Gotcha!
!!!!!

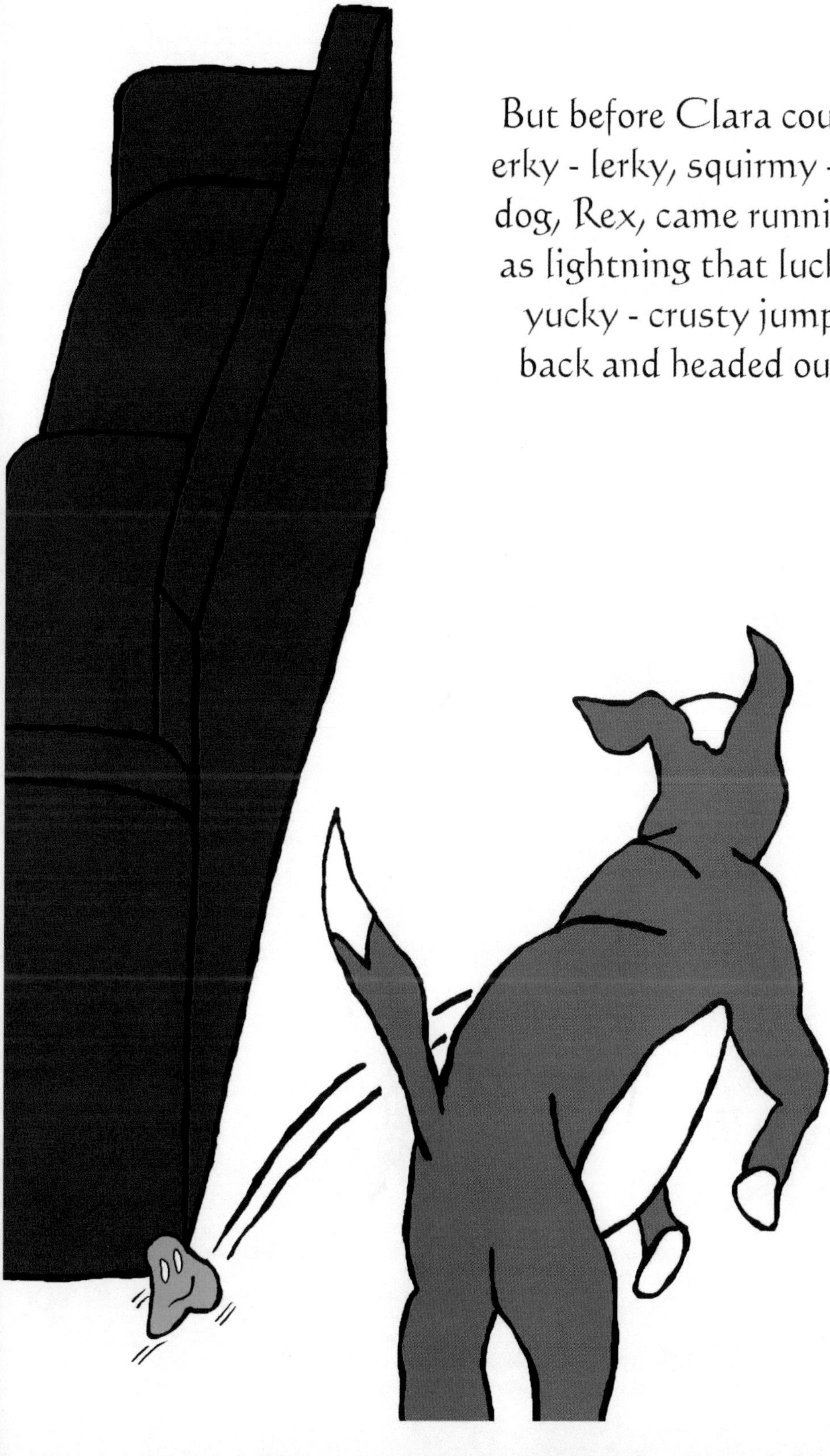

But before Clara could grab the erky - lerky, squirmy - germy, her dog, Rex, came running by. Fast as lightning that lucky - ducky, yucky - crusty jumped on his back and headed out of sight.

Down the hallway they flew. The rinky-dinky, not-a-binky, inky-stinky hanging on for dear life.

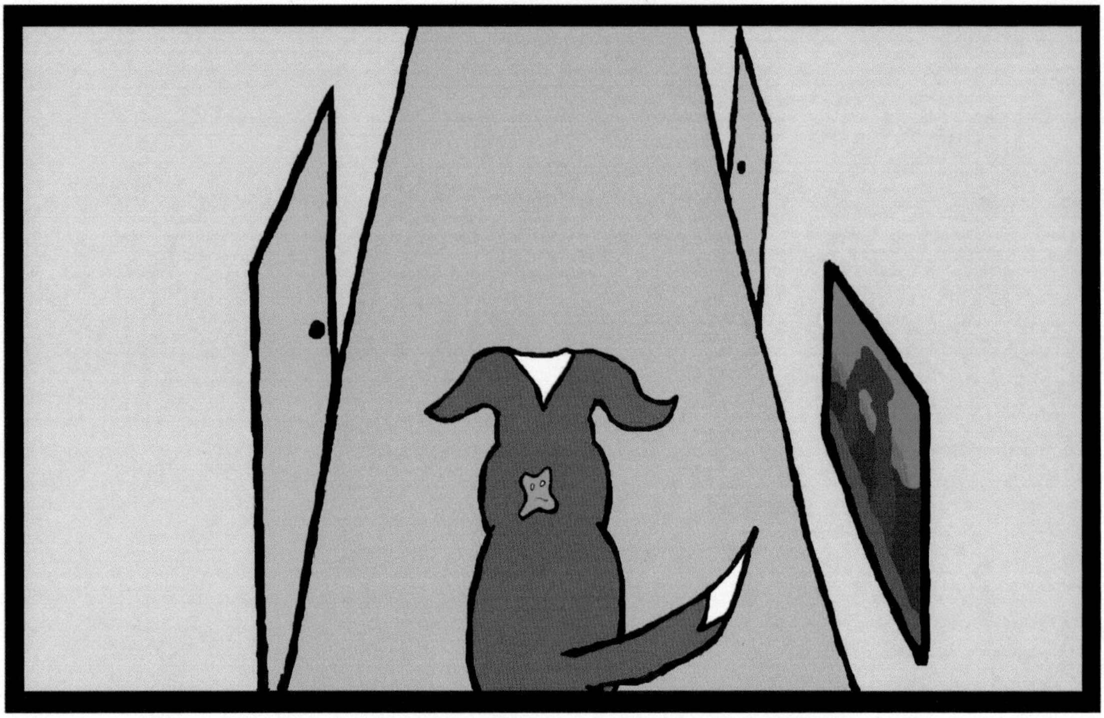

Rex rounded the corner, then skidded to a stop outside the baby's nursey.

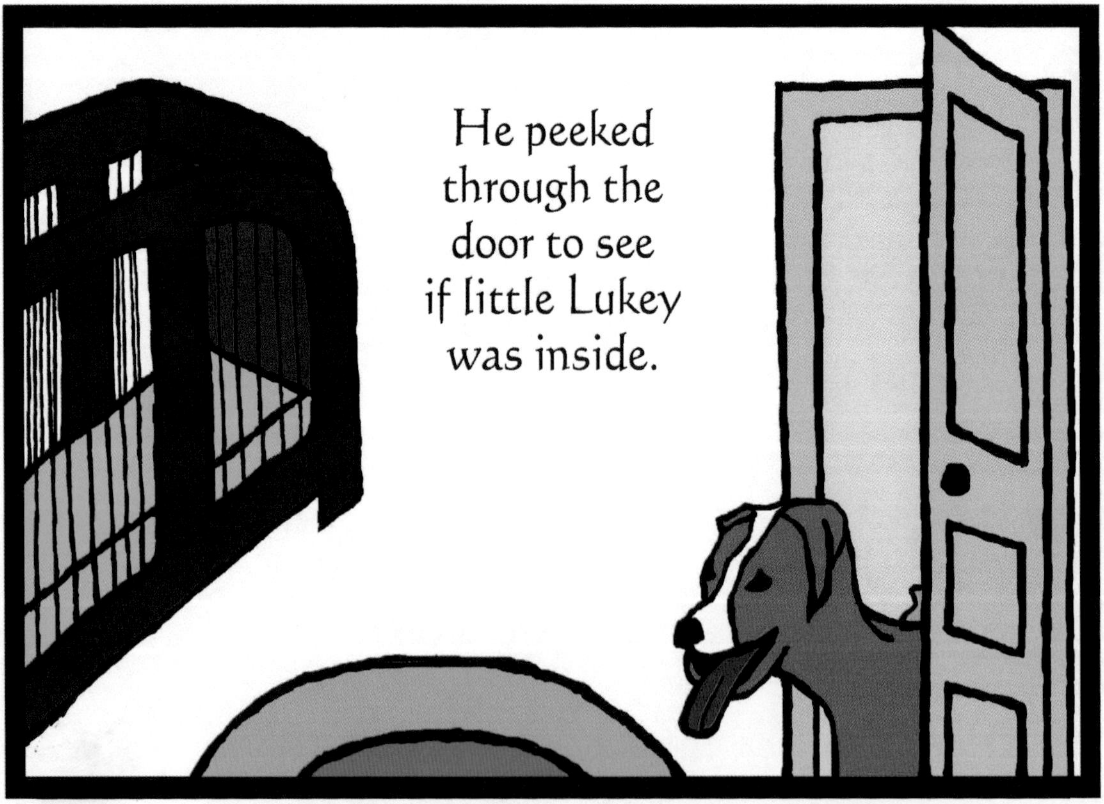
He peeked through the door to see if little Lukey was inside.

What Luck! Baby Lukey was in his room. Rex laid down on the carpet and Luke cuddled up next to him.

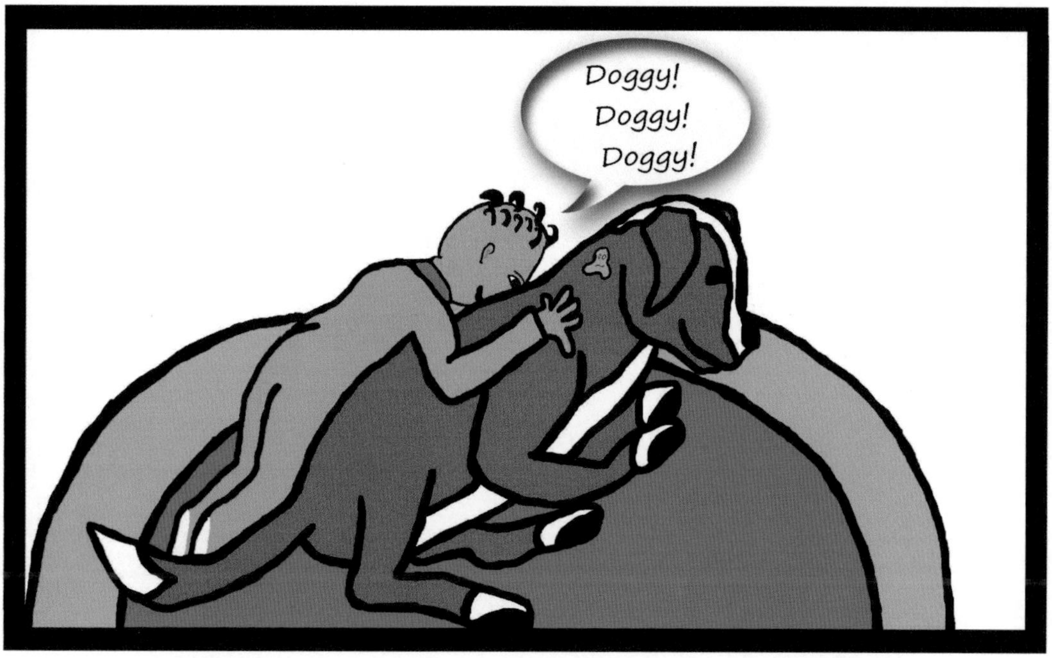
Doggy!
Doggy!
Doggy!

Then that nasty little bogie took the opportunity for slower transporation and jumped onto the top of the baby's head.

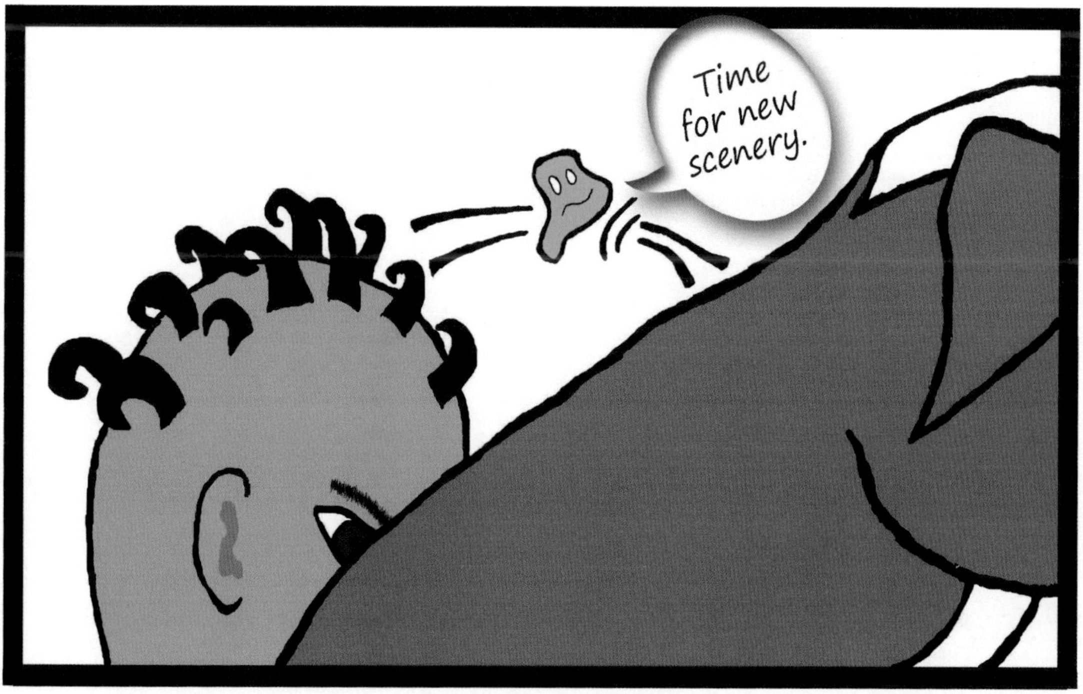
Time for new scenery.

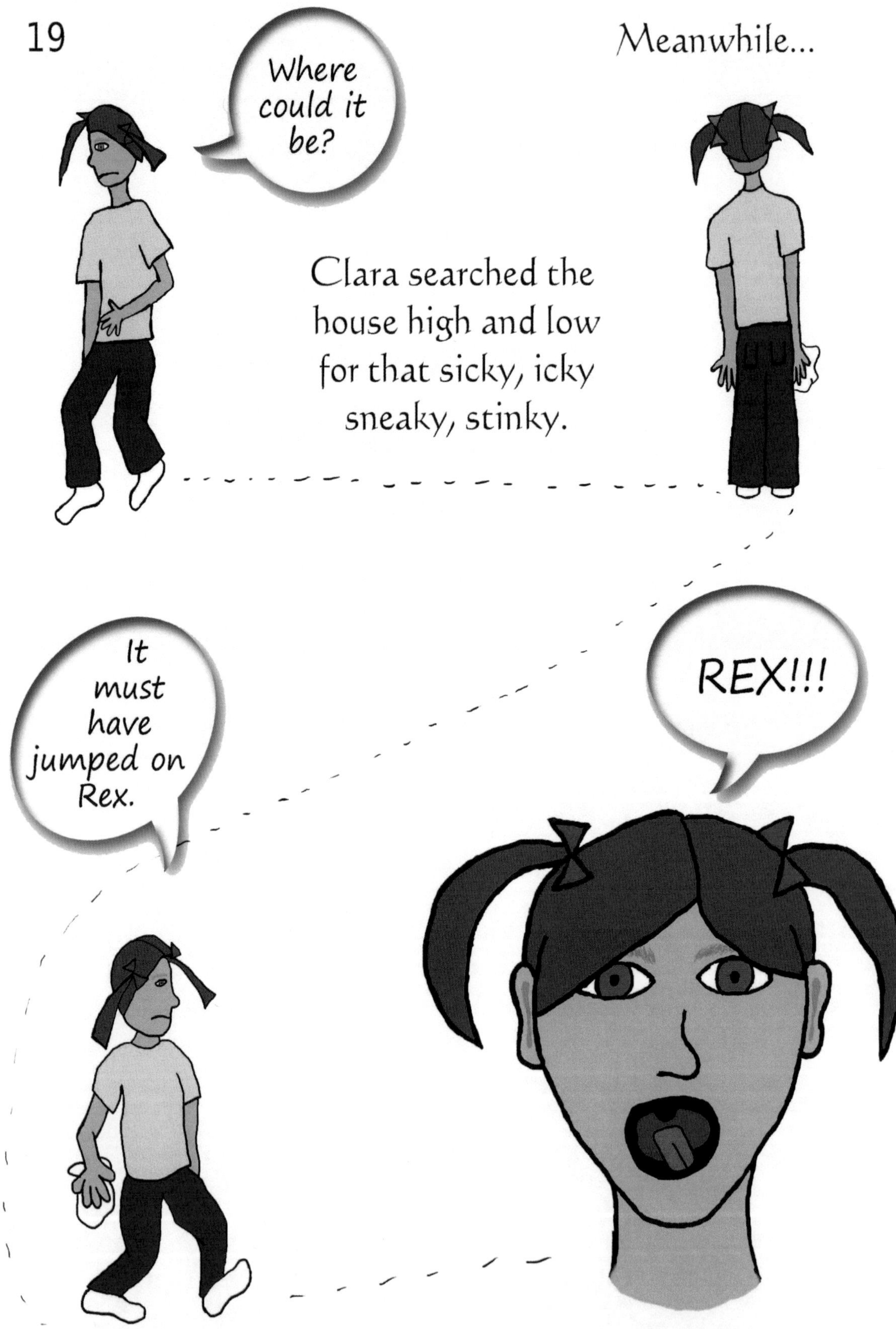
Where could it be?
Meanwhile...
Clara searched the house high and low for that sicky, icky sneaky, stinky.
It must have jumped on Rex.
REX!!!

Hearing his named called, Rex jumped up, accidentally knocked Lukey over, and ran out the door.

WAHHH!!!!
WAHHH!!!!
Can't a booger get a break around here.

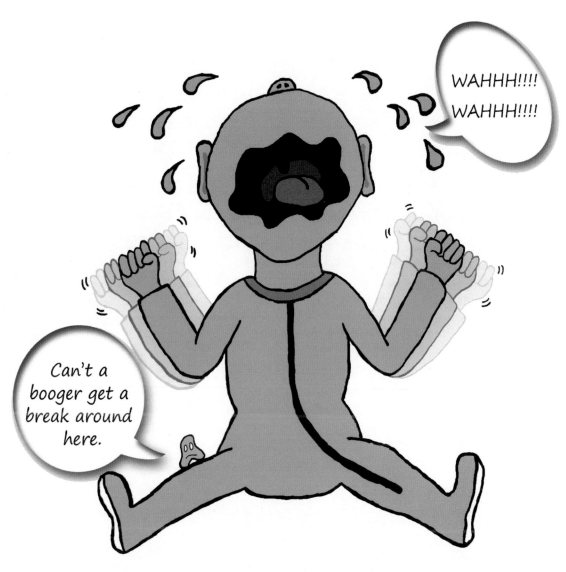

The high pitch wails of the baby sent the creeping, seeping, hot and steaming, ball of snot leaping from its post near Lukey's vocal chords, and down to his knee where the volume was a bit lower.

21 Luke and Clara's mom came running into the nursery to see what had happened.

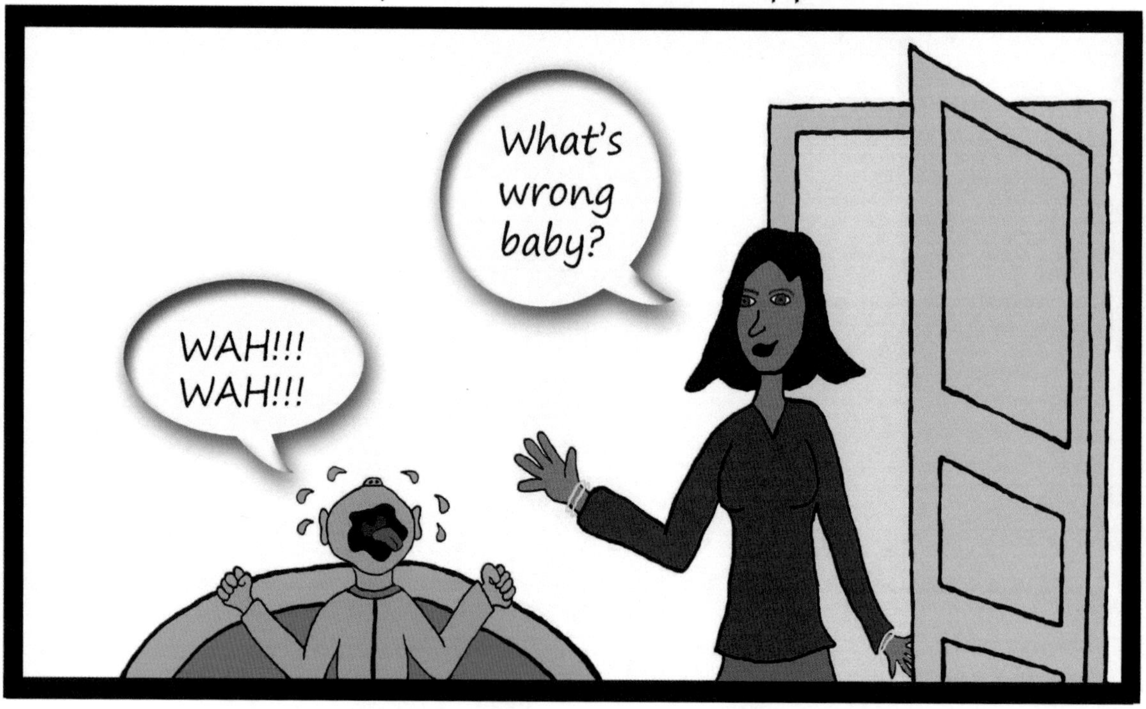
What's wrong baby?
WAH!!! WAH!!!

She scooped Lukey up into her arms and held him tight.

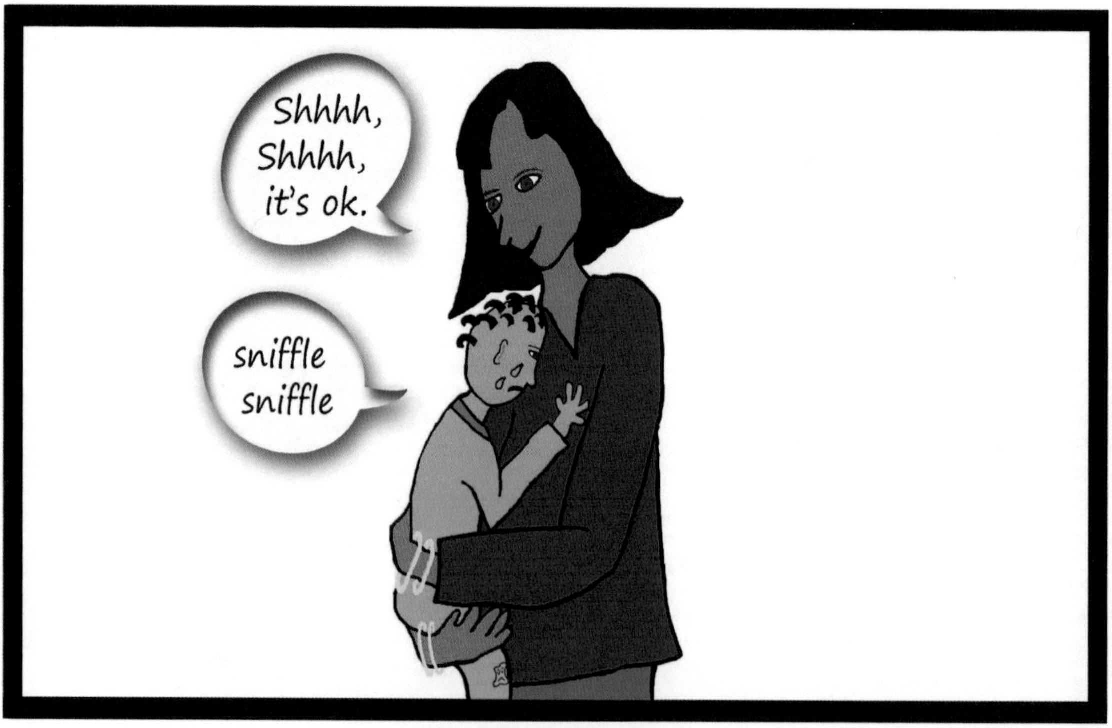
Shhhh, Shhhh, it's ok.
sniffle sniffle

Once again, the slobby, globby, blob of
mucus made a break for it.

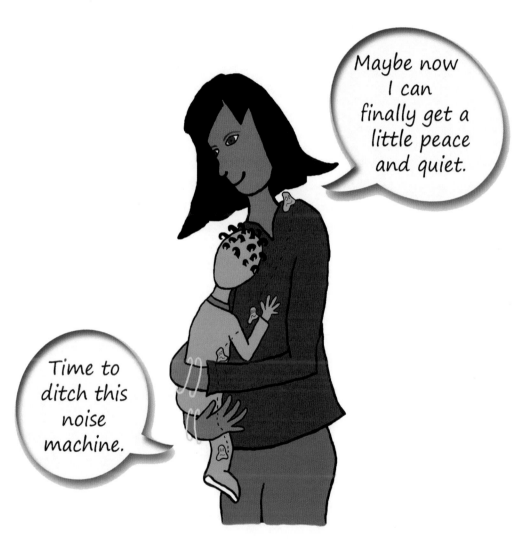

Maybe now
I can
finally get a
little peace
and quiet.

Time to
ditch this
noise
machine.

It climbed up the baby's leg, onto his stomach,
over his arm, and up the mommy's chest,
until settling warm and cozy in the crook
of her neck.

23

Just then, Clara and her dad came bursting into the room.

What's going on in here?
Have you seen a slimey, green, booger anywhere?
What?!?!

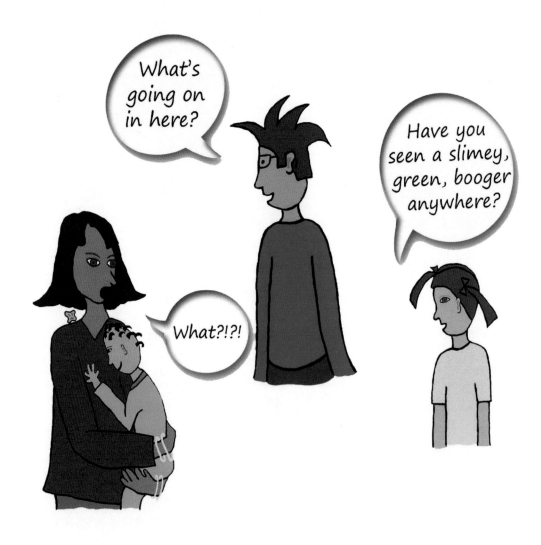

Not taking anymore chances, the smelty - melty - mushy - gushy - oogey - boogey hopped off the mom's shoulder, landed on the crib, and dove for the window.

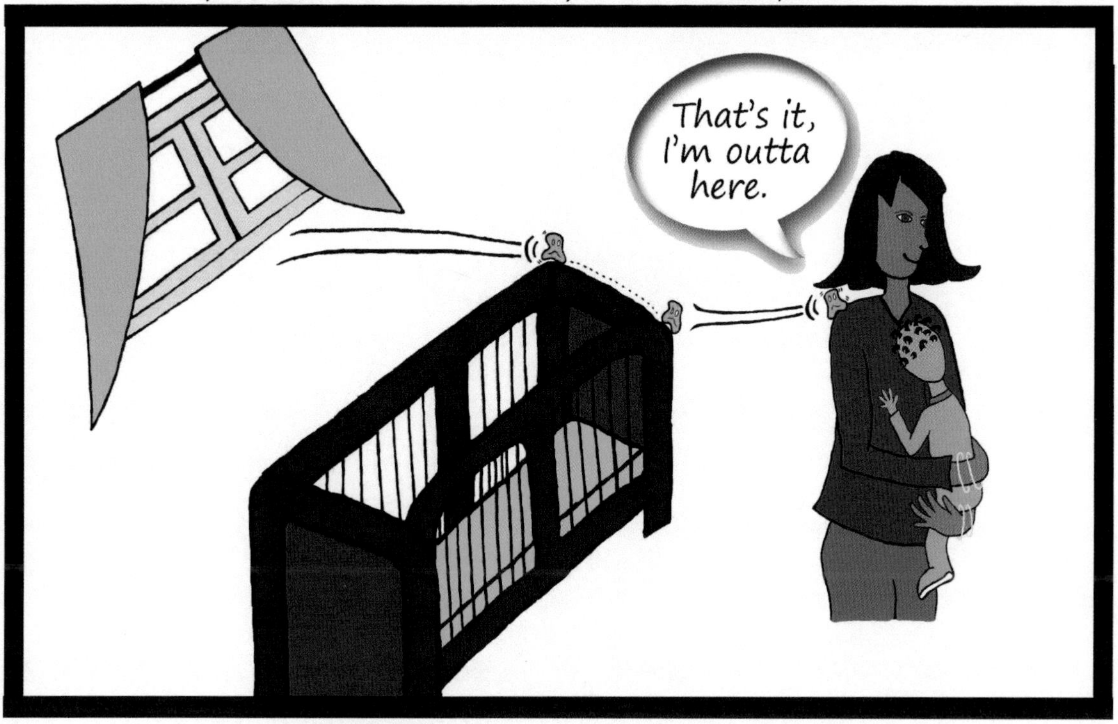
That's it, I'm outta here.

Unfortunately for the boogey, the window was closed.

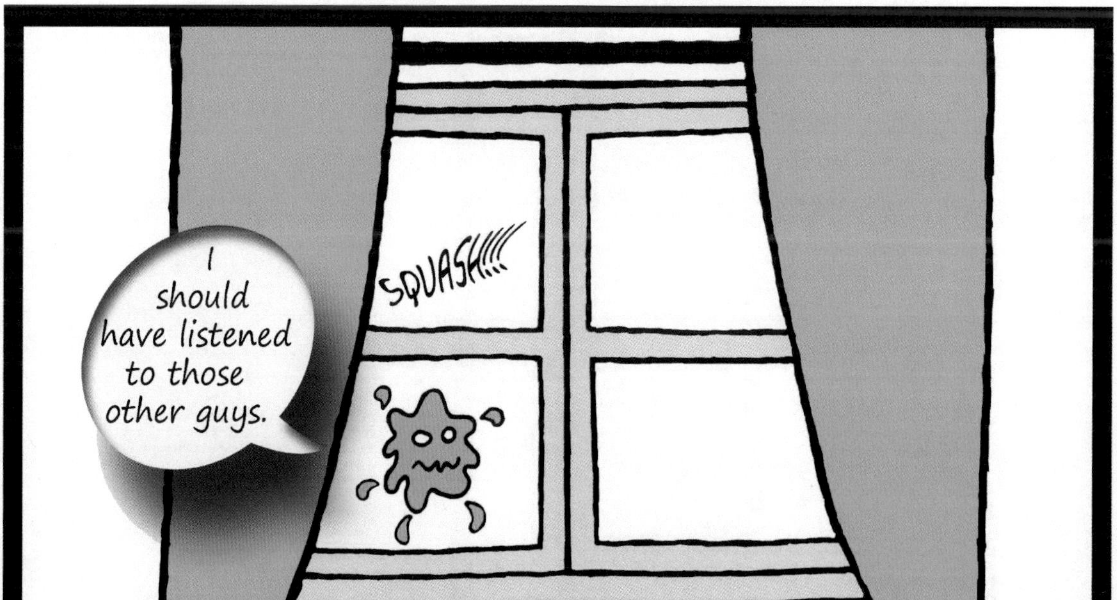
SQUASH!!!!
I should have listened to those other guys.

The sun shone down on the splattered, green and dripping, slimey-snotball, causing it to sparkle against the window.

Look! There it is! On the window!
How'd it get in here?
Germs travel fast.

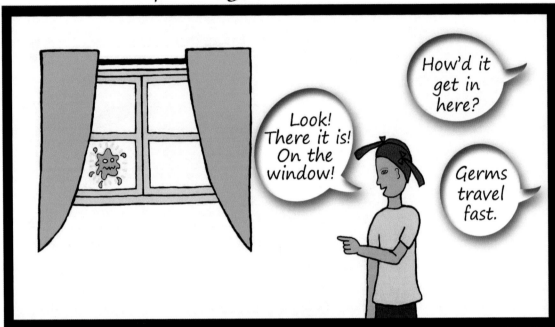

Before it could escape (not that it was in any condition for escaping), Clara rushed over and wiped the glossy, soggy, sloppy, slimeball off the window.

And use some soap!

Then she tossed it into the garbage.
I'm never gonna hear the end of this.

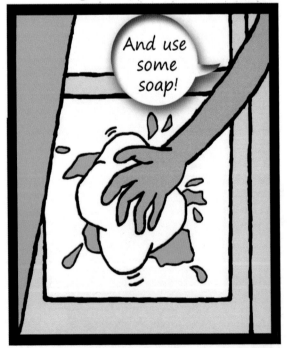

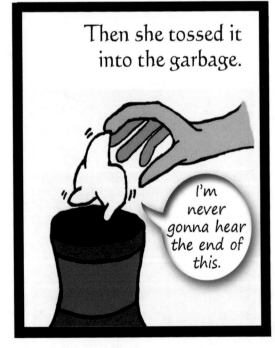

Two days later...

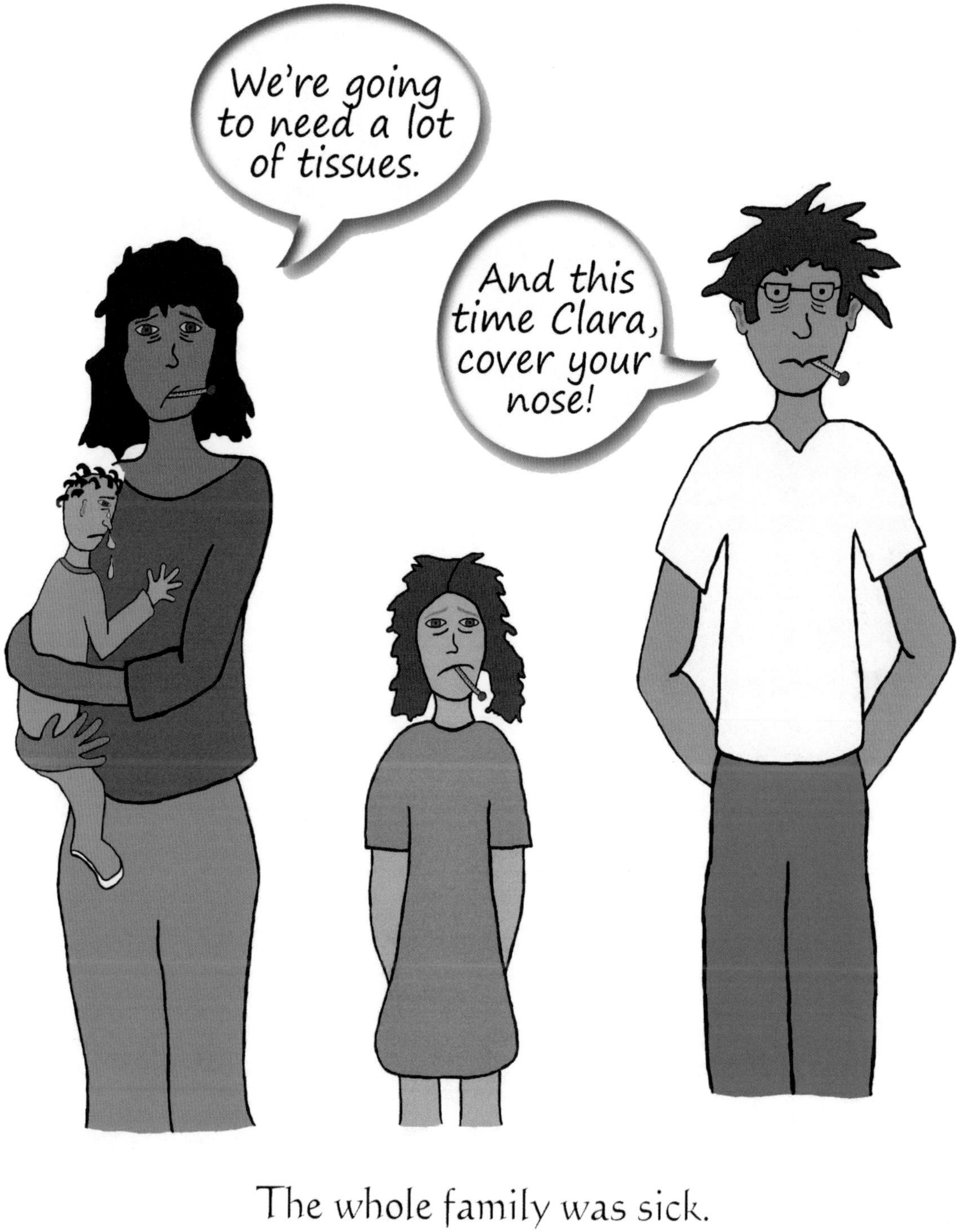
We're going to need a lot of tissues.
And this time Clara, cover your nose!

The whole family was sick.

And the moral of the story is...

Always cover your nose and
mouth when you sneeze.

Or this will be your house...

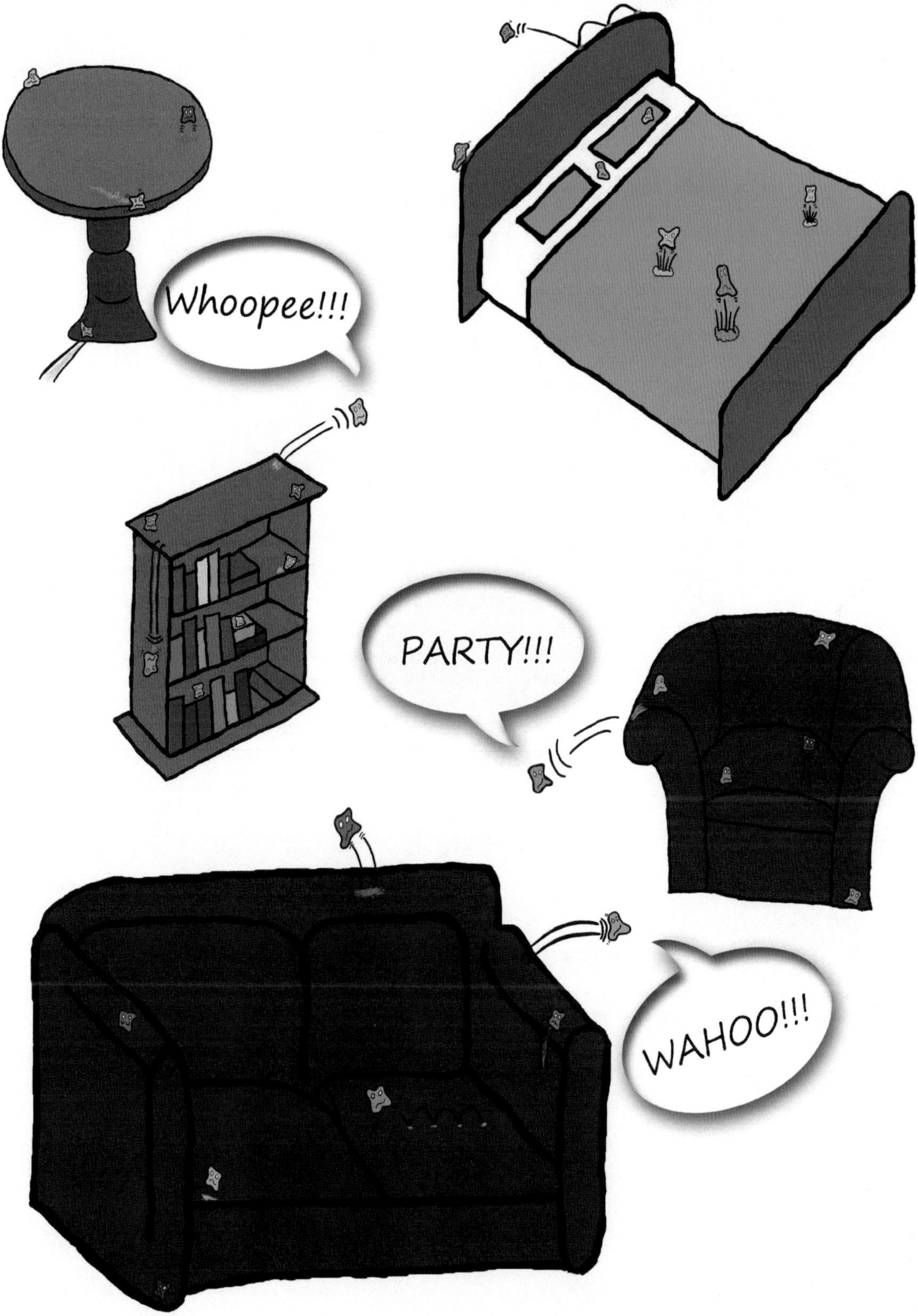
Whoopee!!!
PARTY!!!
WAHOO!!!

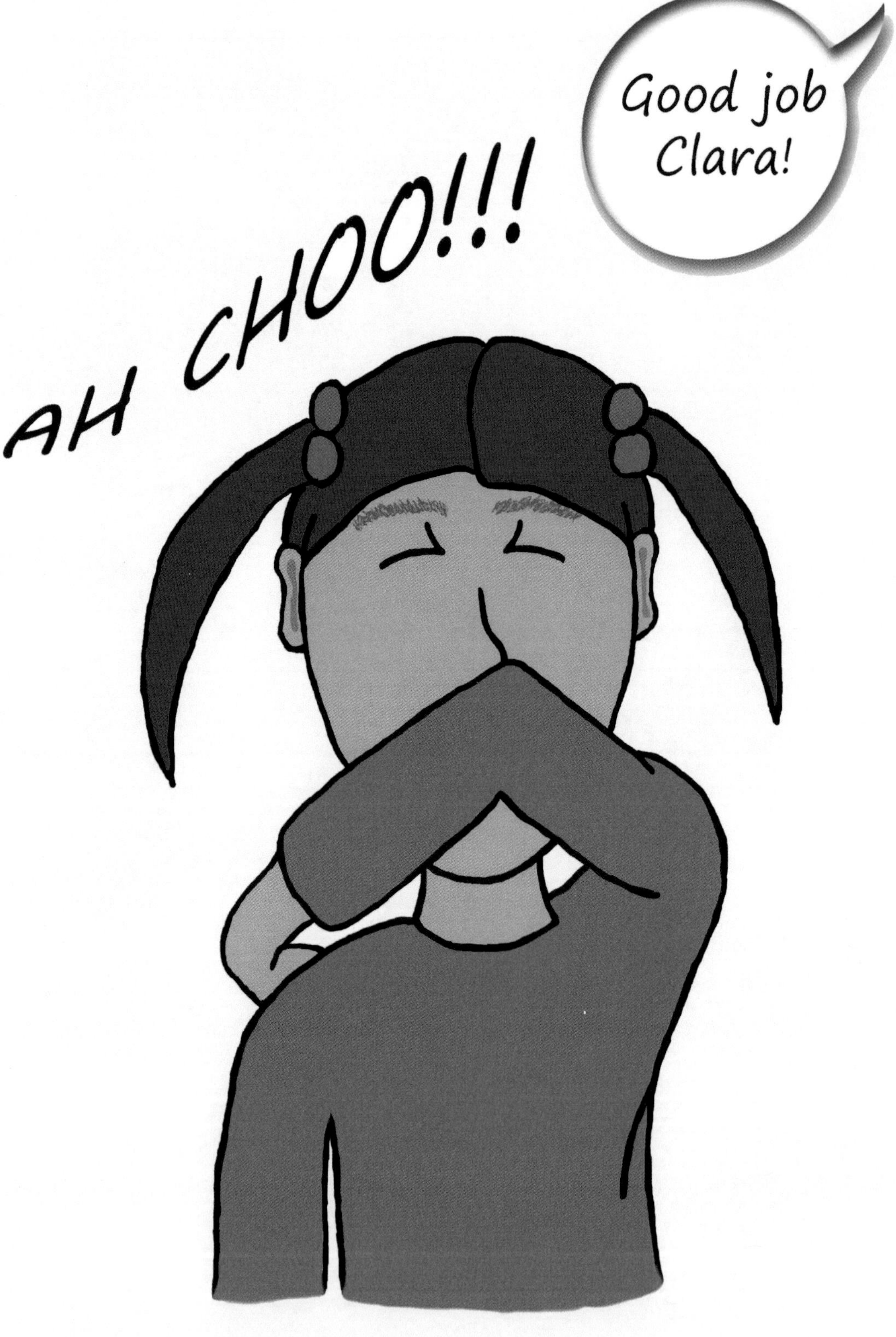
AH CHOO!!!
Good job Clara!

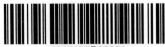

Made in the USA
Charleston, SC
08 September 2015